MW01298114

# Gastric Sleeve Cookbook
## Bundle

# *Gastric Sleeve Cookbook Stage 1*

50 Delicious Herbal & Other Teas, Sugar Free Popsicles & Ice Treats, Broth Recipes You Can Enjoy in Stage 1 Post Weight Loss Surgery Rehabilitation

**Copyright © 2018**

**All Rights Reserved.**

**By Victoria Goode**

Disclaimer Notice

The following is intended for informational purposes only. Patients take all responsibility and must consult their doctor.

# Table of Contents

# Introduction

Congratulations on successfully completing your gastric sleeve surgery! Your new body is going to look great! Now that your surgery is in the past, the hard task of recovery begins. In order to ensure that you recover well and that you maintain the healthy body, you desire you will have to ensure you follow a proper nutrition plan, and it needs to begin right now! Before you can understand how to move on it is vital that you first understand what it is that your body just went through.

## What exactly is Gastric Sleeve Surgery & What does it entail?

Gastric Sleeve or Weight Loss Surgery is a procedure used to help people suffering from obesity to get back to a healthy stage in life by surgically assisting in their weight loss. During the surgery, a portion of the stomach is removed so as to get it smaller (gastric sleeve).

## So, what happens now?

Post your operation; there are four main nutrition goals that you will need to follow. These goals include ensuring you consume the correct amount of protein as this will aid in minimizing the loss of muscle tissue and help to speed up the recovery process. Next would be for you to learn the steps of eating properly as this will assist you in staying healthy in the long run. Thirdly you will need to remember to remain hydrated, ensuring that you drink enough water will be vital to your recovery process. Finally, you will need to ensure that you get the proper nutrients in your body by using supplements for minerals, and vitamins as you won't be able to eat solid food for a while after your surgery.

There will be 4 main stages in terms of food and diet that you will go through post your surgery. Namely:

- Stage 1 – Consuming only Clear Liquids

7

- Stage 2 – Consuming Thicker Liquids & Smooth Foods
- Stage 3 – Consuming Soft Pureed Foods
- Stage 4 – Consuming Regular Foods

This Gastric Sleeve Cookbook will focus on Stage 1 of your post gastric sleeve surgery recovery process helping you to understand what you can eat. So, let's explore Stage 1 of the recovery process a bit more so that you can fully understand what is expected at this stage.

## _Stage I – Consuming only Clear Liquids_

This stage generally encompasses the first 7 days after your surgery, however, in all cases, it may be different. In this stage of the recovery, it is recommended that you stick to a diet filled with clear liquids. Sticking to clear liquids will allow your body to heal without disruption from the foods that your stomach would need to digest. You will, of course, need to take it slowly at first, so it's recommended, to begin with trying to drink about two ounces of liquid at a time as often as every 30 minutes. After which based on how you feel you can slowly increase your intake to up to eight ounces per hour. It is important to note that eating or drinking may cause discomfort so try to drink slowly, sip and not gulp.

Remember hydration is vital in this stage of recovery so try to consume at least 48 ounces to 64 ounces of liquid per day.

## _Here are some Important Tips to Remember:_

- Try to avoid drinks with too much sugar, caffeine or carbonation as they can disrupt the healing process by causing side effects.
- Be sure to sip and not gulp as drinking in small portions makes it better for your body to readjust.
- Drinking a lot of liquids is of utmost importance, recording your daily liquid intake may help you greatly in avoiding dehydration.

So now that you know a bit more about Gastric Sleeve Surgery let's explore a bit more about what exactly you can eat within this clear liquid the only stage. In this Gastric Sleeve Cookbook, you will be exposed to 50 simple yet tasty recipes that are all easy on the stomach. Without further ado, let's get started.

# _Herbal & Other Teas_

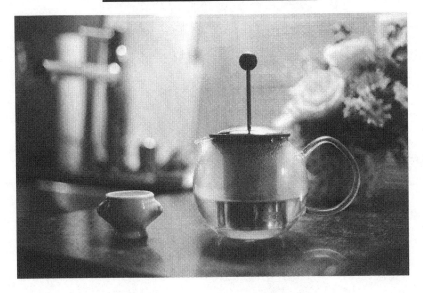

# Peppermint Tea

This tea is said to help with abdominal gas and bloating.

Preparation time: 37 minutes
Yield: 4 servings

Ingredients
- Peppermint Leaf (1/2 cup, dried)
- Water (4 cups, hot)

Directions
1. Set your water on to boil. Once boiling add in your peppermint leaves and remove from heat.
2. Cover and let rest for at least 5 minutes.
3. Strain, serve and enjoy

Macros per Serving & Nutrition Facts
- Calories 34.2
- Total Fat 0.0 g
- Carbohydrate 9.1 g
- Protein 0.1g

# Pecan Tea

Yet another warm beverage is perfect for the early mornings.

Preparation Time: 20 minutes
Serving: 2

Ingredients
- Pecans (5 tablespoons, grounded)
- Cinnamon (1 tsp.)
- Water (1 cup)

Directions

1. Heat a cup of water in a saucepan and then stir in your remaining ingredients.
2. Serve hot.

Macros per Serving & Nutrition Facts
- Calories 40
- Total Fat 3.58 g
- Carbohydrate 1.4 g
- Protein 1.51 g

# *Ginger Tea*

This tea has been known to help curb an upset stomach, nausea and even subdue vomiting.

Preparation time: 15 minutes
Yield: 2 serving

Ingredients
- Gingerroot (3 tsp., grated))
- Boiling Water (3 cups)

Directions
1. Combine your ingredients together and allow to rest, covered for at least 10 minutes.
2. Serve and Enjoy!

Macros per Serving & Nutrition Facts
- Calories 26.8
- Total Fat 0.0 g
- Carbohydrate 6.8 g
- Protein 0.1 g

# Orange Vanilla Tea

Classic Orange tea with a hint of vanilla, for a surprise.

Preparation time: 11 minutes
Yields: 2.5 Cups

Ingredients
- Water (1/4 cup)
- Oranges (2, medium, peeled, sliced)
- Vanilla Extract (1/4 tsp.)

Directions
1. Pour all your ingredients into a saucepan and allow to come to a boil.
2. Remove from heat and let rest for about 5 minutes.
3. Strain, serve and enjoy!

Macros per Serving & Nutrition Facts
- Calories 60
- Total Fat 0.0 g
- Carbohydrate 14 g
- Protein 1g

# Peanut Tea

Get something warm in the morning.

Preparation Time: 20 minutes
Serving: 2

Ingredients
- Peanut (5 tablespoons, grounded)
- Cinnamon (1 tsp.)
- Water (1 cup)

Directions
1. Heat a cup of water in a saucepan and then stir in your remaining ingredients.
2. Serve hot.

Macros per Serving & Nutrition Facts
- Calories 40
- Total Fat 3.58 g
- Carbohydrate 1.4 g
- Protein 1.51 g

## *Red Apple and Carrot Tea*

This tea is best for chronic constipation. Make it and drink 1 glass daily for better results.

Preparation time: 6 minutes
Yield: 3 servings

Ingredients
- 1 cup red apples, peeled, chunks
- 2 carrots, sliced
- ½ cup lychee, seeded
- 2 cups water

Directions
1. Blend apples with carrots, lychee, and water.
2. Pour all your ingredients into a saucepan and allow to come to a boil.
3. Remove from heat and let rest for about 5 minutes.
4. Strain, serve and enjoy!

Macros per Serving & Nutrition Facts
- Calories 184
- Total Fat 0.0 g
- Carbohydrate 44.6g
- Protein 1g

# Orange Carrot Tea

This recipe gives a rich blend of both orange and carrot. If you love a strong citrusy drink, you will love this!

Yields: 5 cups
Time Needed: 11 minutes

Ingredients
- Oranges (4, peeled, halved)
- Carrots (12 oz., diced)
- Water (4 Cups)

Directions
1. Pour all your ingredients into the Vitamix and secure the lid.
2. Pour all your ingredients into a saucepan and allow to come to a boil.
3. Remove from heat and let rest for about 5 minutes.
4. Strain, serve and enjoy!

Macros per Serving & Nutrition Facts
- Calories 93
- Total Fat 0.4 g
- Carbohydrate 22 g
- Protein 2.2g


# Almond Tea

Begin your day with a splash of almond tea.

Serving: 2
Preparation Time: 20 minutes

Ingredients
- Almond Powder (5 tablespoons)
- Cinnamon (1 tsp.)

- Water (1 cup)

Directions
1. Heat a cup of water in a saucepan and then stir in your remaining ingredients.
2. Serve hot.

Macros per Serving & Nutrition Facts
- Calories 40
- Total Fat 3.58 g
- Carbohydrate 1.4 g
- Protein 1.51 g

# *Rooibos Tea*

Packed with vitamin C, as well as other antioxidants and minerals, this tea aids immensely in the recovery process.

Preparation time: 30 minutes
Yield: 4 servings

Ingredients
- Rooibos (1/2 cup)
- Water (4 cups, hot)

Directions
1. Set your water on to boil. Once boiling add in your rooibos pieces and remove from heat.
2. Cover and let rest for at least 15 minutes.
3. Strain, serve and enjoy

Macros per Serving & Nutrition Facts
- Calories 1
- Total Fat 0.0 g
- Carbohydrate 0.1 g
- Protein 0 g

# Chamomile Tea

This tea can be used as a natural sedative as it calms the nerves. It is also said to aid in the digestion process which makes it a brilliant option during stage 1 recovery.

Preparation time: 10 minutes
Yield: 2 servings

Ingredients
- Chamomile Flowers (2 tbsp.)
- Water (2 cups)

Directions
1. Set your water on to boil. Once boiling add in your chamomile and remove from heat.
2. Cover and let rest for at least 5 minutes.
3. Strain, serve and enjoy

Macros per Serving & Nutrition Facts
- Calories 1
- Total Fat 0 g
- Sodium 4.7 mg
- Carbohydrate 0.1 g
- Protein 0.0g

# Lemon Balm Tea

This tea is great for relaxation.

Preparation time: 20 minutes
Yield: 5 servings

Ingredients
- Lemon Balm (1 cup)
- Water (5 cups)

- Lemon Zest (1 tbsp.)

Directions
1. Set your water on to boil. Once boiling add in your lemon balm, and zest then remove from heat.
2. Cover and let rest for at least 10 minutes.
3. Strain, serve and enjoy

Macros per Serving & Nutrition Facts
- Calories 13.3
- Total Fat 0 g
- Carbohydrate 3.6 g
- Protein 0.0g

# *Dandelion Tea*

Here is a tea that works to cleanse your livers, and aids in bile production which is vital in the digestion process.

Preparation time: 10 minutes
Yield: 2 servings

Ingredients
- Dandelion Flowers (2 tbsp.)
- Water (2 cups)

Directions
1. Set your water on to boil. Once boiling add in your dandelion and remove from heat.
2. Cover and let rest for at least 5 minutes.
3. Strain, serve and enjoy

Macros per Serving & Nutrition Facts
- Calories 8
- Total Fat 0 g
- Carbohydrate 0.0 g
- Protein 0.0g

# Hibiscus Tea

Hibiscus tea is said to keep high cholesterol and high blood pressure at bay.

Preparation time: 10 minutes
Yield: 2 servings

Ingredients
- Hibiscus Flowers (4 tbsp.)
- Water (2 cups)

Directions
1. Set your water on to boil. Once boiling add in your hibiscus and remove from heat.
2. Cover and let rest for at least 5 minutes.
3. Strain, serve and enjoy

Macros per Serving & Nutrition Facts
- Calories 9
- Total Fat 0.7 g
- Carbohydrate 0 g
- Protein 0.4 g

# Green Tea

Green tea carries a myriad of health benefits, including fat loss, improving brain function, and even lowering the risk of cancer.

Preparation time: 20 minutes
Yield: 2 servings

Ingredients
- Camellia Sinensis Leaves (4 tbsp., fresh)
- Water (2 cups)

Directions

1.  Set your water on to boil. Once boiling add in your Camellia and remove from heat.
2.  Cover and let rest for at least 10 minutes.
3.  Strain, serve and enjoy

Macros per Serving & Nutrition Facts

- Calories 10
- Total Fat 0.1 g
- Saturated Fat 0.0 g
- Carbohydrate 0 g
- Protein 0 g

# _Sugar Free Popsicles & Ice Treat_

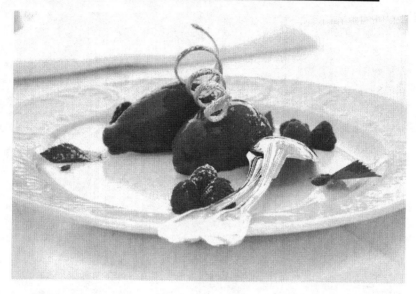

# Watermelon sorbet

Watermelon sorbet tastes refreshing on the pallet.

Serves: 6
Time: 5 minutes

Ingredients:
- 4 ½ cups ice cubes, crushed
- ½lb Melon, cubed
- 1 tablespoon grated orange zest

Directions:
1. Place all ingredients in a blender.
2. Blend the ingredients for 30 seconds.
3. Serve immediately.

NB: We suggest that you make the sorbet in batches.

Macros per Serving & Nutrition Facts
- Calories 231.1
- Total Fat 0.2 g
- Carbohydrate 59.6 g
- Protein 0.6 g

# Banana Icy Pops

This recipe is great for in the morning when you need a pick me up.

Serving Size: 8
Overall time: 4 hours and 30 minutes

Ingredients:
- Boiling water (1 cup)
- Fruit-flavored Jell-O (1 package)
- Banana (1)
- Plain yogurt (1 cup)

Directions:
1. Add all the ingredients in a blender. Blend everything thing until it is smooth.
2. Put mixture into a popsicle mold or an in a plastic cup.
3. Place in a freezer until hard.
4. Serve and enjoy!

Macros per Serving & Nutrition Facts
- Calories 93
- Total Fat 0.4 g
- Carbohydrate 22 g
- Protein 2.2g

# *Kiwi Sorbet*

Cool your digestive tract with this delicious sugar free sorbet.

Serves: 6
Time: 5 minutes

Ingredients:
- 4 ½ cups ice cubes, crushed
- ½lb Kiwi, chopped
- 1 tablespoon grated orange zest

Directions:
1. Place all ingredients in a blender.
2. Blend the ingredients for 30 seconds.
3. Serve immediately.
NB: We suggest that you make the sorbet in batches.

Macros per Serving & Nutrition Facts
- Calories 105.5
- Total Fat 0.3 g
- Saturated Fat 0.0 g
- Carbohydrate 26.7 g
- Protein 0.6 g

# Raspberry Icy Pops

If you love raspberry, then give these sugar free popsicles a go.

Serving Size: 8
Overall time: 4 hours and 30 minutes

Ingredients:
- Boiling water (1 cup)
- Jell-O (1 package, raspberry)
- Raspberries (1 cup, fresh)
- Plain yogurt (1 cup)

Directions:
1. Add all the ingredients in a blender. Blend everything thing until it is smooth.
2. Put mixture into a popsicle mold and place to freeze until frozen.
3. Serve and enjoy!

Macros per Serving & Nutrition Facts
- Calories 1.3
- Total Fat 0.0 g
- Carbohydrate 0.4 g
- Protein 0.0 g

# Strawberry Icy Pops

These popsicles are naturally sweet and acts as a good treat in stage 1 recovery.

Serving Size: 8
Overall time: 4 hours and 30 minutes

Ingredients:
- Boiling water (1 cup)

- Fruit-flavored Jell-O (1 package)
- Strawberries (1 cup)
- Plain yogurt (1 cup)

Directions:
1. Add all the ingredients in a blender. Blend everything thing until it is smooth.
2. Put mixture into a popsicle mold or an in a plastic cup.
3. Place in a freezer until hard.
4. Serve and enjoy!

Macros per Serving & Nutrition Facts
- Calories 90
- Total Fat 1.42 g
- Carbohydrate 18.49 g
- Protein 0.71 g

# *Fruit Infused Water*

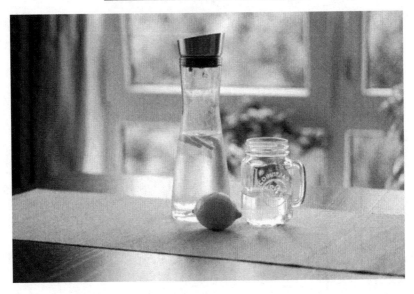

# Lemon, Mint & Cucumber Infused Water

This mix is perfect for flushing our bodies of unwanted toxins. As an added bonus, the lemons in this recipe aids in digestion while the cucumber helps to keep you refreshed and hydrated.

Makes: 48 fl. oz.
Time: 5 minutes + chilling time

Ingredients:
- 6 cups water
- 1 grapefruit, sliced
- 1 orange, sliced
- ½ cup cucumber slices

Directions
1. Combine all the ingredients in a pitcher.
2. Refrigerate for 2 hours or overnight.
3. Serve in the morning and drink through the day.

Macros per Serving & Nutrition Facts
- Calories 1.3
- Total Fat 0.0 g
- Carbohydrate 0.4 g
- Protein 0.0 g

# Citrus & Mint Infused Water

Tasty and refreshing infused water that helps to promote weight loss.
Makes: 64 Fl.oz.
Time: 5 minutes + chilling time

Ingredients:
- ½ red grapefruit, segmented
- 2 mint leaves

- ½ lemon, sliced
- 1 cucumber, sliced
- ½ lime sliced
- ½ gallon spring water

Directions
1. Wash and prepare the ingredients.
2. Place all the ingredients in a pitcher.
3. Refrigerate for 2 hours.
4. Serve after.

Macros per Serving & Nutrition Facts
- Calories 2
- Total Fat 0.0 g
- Carbohydrate 0.4 g
- Protein 0.0 g

## *Pineapple and Mango Water*

This juice will help you to boost your stamina.

Makes: 64 Fl.oz.
Time: 5 minutes + chilling time

Ingredients
- 1 cup pineapple slices
- 1 cup ripe mango, chunks
- 10 cups water
- ½ teaspoon protein powder
- 1-inch ginger sliced, peeled

Directions
1. Transfer all ingredients into a pitcher and place to chill for at least an hour.
2. Pour into serving glasses and serve.

Macros per Serving & Nutrition Facts
- Calories 10
- Total Fat 0.0 g
- Carbohydrate 12 g
- Protein 0.0 g

## Honeydew & Kiwi Infused Water

If you love tropical fruits, this may just be the mix for you.

Makes: 64 Fl.oz.
Time: 5 minutes + chilling time

Ingredients:
- 1 kiwi, peeled and sliced
- 2 cups honeydew melon, chopped
- 10 cups Water

Directions
1. In a pitcher combine the fruits.
2. Fill to the top with water.
3. Refrigerate for 1 hour before serving.

Macros per Serving & Nutrition Facts
- Calories 12
- Total Fat 0.0 g
- Carbohydrate 4.4 g
- Protein 0.0 g

## Sweet and Sour Lychee Infused Water

This is a unique recipe, make it and enjoy with your family members.

Makes: 64 Fl.oz.
Time: 5 minutes + chilling time

Ingredients
- 1 cup lychees, peeled, seeded
- 1 tbsp. ginger powder
- 10 cups water
- 3 tablespoons lemon juice

Directions
1. Combine all your ingredients in a pitcher.
2. Refrigerate for 1 hour before serving.

Macros per Serving & Nutrition Facts
- Calories 2
- Total Fat 0.0 g
- Carbohydrate 31g
- Protein 0.0 g

## *Kiwi and Kale Detox Water*

Rich with calcium and omega-3 antioxidant.

Makes: 64 Fl.oz.
Time: 5 minutes + chilling time

Ingredients
- 4 kiwis, sliced
- 5 kale leaves
- 10 cups cold water

Directions
1. Combine all your ingredients in a pitcher.
2. Refrigerate for 1 hour before serving.

Macros per Serving & Nutrition Facts
- Calories 1.7
- Total Fat 0.0g
- Carbohydrate 8 g
- Protein 17 g

# Honeydew & Kiwi Infused Water

If you love tropical fruits, this may just be the mix for you.

Makes: 64 fl.oz.
Time: 5 minutes + chilling time

Ingredients:
- 1 kiwi, peeled and sliced
- 2 cups honeydew melon, chopped
- 10 cups Water

Directions
1. In a pitcher combine the fruits.
2. Fill to the top with water.
3. Refrigerate for 1 hour before serving.

Macros per Serving & Nutrition Facts
- Calories 1.3
- Total Fat 0.0 g
- Carbohydrate 0.4 g
- Protein 0.0 g

# Watermelon and Lemon Water

Drink this juice to prevent the diseases like asthma, clogging and airway.

Preparation time: 10 minutes
Yield: 2 servings

Ingredients
- 3 cups watermelon, chunks, seeded
- 3 tablespoons lemon juice
- 2-3 mint leaves
- 1 pinch salt

- 10 cups water

Directions
1. Combine all your ingredients in a pitcher.
2. Refrigerate for 1 hour before serving.

Macros per Serving & Nutrition Facts
- Calories 105.1
- Total Fat 1.4 g
- Carbohydrate 24.6 g
- Protein 2.1 g

# *Mango & Ginger Infused Water*

Another refreshing drink that boosts the metabolism and promotes weight loss

Makes: 64 fl.oz.
Time: 5 minutes + chilling time

Ingredients:
- 1 cup diced mango
- 1-inch ginger, peeled and sliced
- 2 cups ice
- Water, to top off

Directions
1. Peel and slice the ginger in 3-4 coin size slices.
2. Transfer the ginger into a pitcher along with mango.
3. Top with 2 cups ice and fill with water.
4. Refrigerate for 3 hours.
5. Serve after.

Macros per Serving & Nutrition Facts
- Calories 1.3
- Total Fat 0.0 g
- Carbohydrate 0.4 g
- Protein 0.0 g

# Lavender & Blueberry Infused Water

Refreshing, healthy and delicious!

Makes: 64 fl. oz.
Time: 5 minutes + chilling time

Ingredients:
- 8 cups water
- 1-pint fresh blueberries
- 1 tablespoon lavender flowers

Directions
1. Mix all your ingredients in a large pitcher.
2. Stir gently and refrigerate for 1 hour.
3. Strain and serve with ice.

Macros per Serving & Nutrition Facts
- Calories 1.3
- Total Fat 0.0 g
- Carbohydrate 0.4 g
- Protein 0.0 g

# Grapefruit, Orange & Cucumber Infused Water

This mix is perfect for flushing our bodies of unwanted toxins.

Makes: 48 fl. oz.
Time: 5 minutes + chilling time

Ingredients:
- 6 cups water
- 1 grapefruit, sliced
- 1 orange, sliced
- ½ cup cucumber slices

## Directions

1. Combine all the ingredients in a pitcher.
2. Refrigerate for 2 hours or overnight.
3. Serve in the morning and drink through the day.

Macros per Serving & Nutrition Facts
- Calories 1.3
- Total Fat 0.0 g
- Carbohydrate 0.4 g
- Protein 0.0 g

# *Pina Colada Infused Water*

This recipe offers a play on the flavors of Pina Colada while maintaining a variety of health benefits.

Makes: 48 fl. oz.
Time: 5 minutes + chilling time

Ingredients:
- 1 cup peeled and thinly sliced pineapple
- 2 cups ice
- 6 cups Coconut Water

Directions

1. Pour out your pineapple into a large pitcher.
2. Top with ice.
3. Pour in water to the top and cover.
4. Refrigerate for 1 hour before serving.

Macros per Serving & Nutrition Facts
- Calories 1.3
- Total Fat 0.0 g
- Carbohydrate 0.4 g
- Protein 0.0 g

# Orange & Blueberry Infused Water

A tasty blend that does well for detoxing.

Makes: 48 fl.oz.
Time: 5 minutes + chilling time

Ingredients:
- 2 oranges, cut into wedges
- 1 cup blueberries
- 6 cups water

Directions
1. Combine all ingredients in a pitcher.
2. Cover and allow to chill for a minimum of 2 hours or overnight.
3. Serve after.

Macros per Serving & Nutrition Facts
- Calories 1.3
- Total Fat 0.0 g
- Carbohydrate 0.4 g
- Protein 0.0 g

# Coconut and Blueberry Infused Water

This delicious blueberry juice with coconut water is most suitable for summer.

Makes: 64 Fl.oz.
Time: 5 minutes + chilling time

Ingredients
- 3 cup blueberries
- 10 cups coconut water

Directions
1. Combine all ingredients in a pitcher.
2. Cover and allow to chill for a minimum of 2 hours or overnight.
3. Serve after.

Macros per Serving & Nutrition Facts
- Calories 9
- Total Fat 1.42 g
- Carbohydrate 8.49 g
- Protein 0.71 g

# Raspberry & Orange Infused Water

This recipe offers the sweetness of the raspberries and the tanginess of the oranges; together it is simply delicious.

Makes: 48fl. oz.
Time: 5 minutes + chilling time

Ingredients:
- 2 mandarin oranges, cut into wedges
- ½ cup raspberries
- 6 cups water

Directions
1. Place all the ingredients into a pitcher.
2. Cover and allow to chill for a minimum of 2 hours or overnight.
3. Serve after.

Macros per Serving & Nutrition Facts
- Calories 1.3
- Total Fat 0.0 g
- Carbohydrate 0.4 g

# Strawberry, Lemon & Basil Infused Water

This mix has become very popular in spas over the years because it promotes healthy skin, detox and even helps in boosting the metabolism.

Makes: 32 fl.oz.
Time: 5 minutes + chilling time

Ingredients:
- 6 strawberries, hulled and sliced
- ½ lemon, sliced
- 1 small handful basil, scrunched
- 4 cups water

Directions
1. In a pitcher combine all ingredients.
2. Cover and allow to chill for a minimum of 2 hours or overnight.
3. Serve after or drink through the day.

Macros per Serving & Nutrition Facts
- Calories 1.3
- Total Fat 0.0 g
- Carbohydrate 0.4 g
- Protein 0.0 g

# Ginger Greens Infused Water

Vegetable water is often swallow, but this recipe aims to correct that by providing the perfect blend of vegetables and ginger.

Makes: 64 fl. Oz.
Time: 5 minutes + chilling time

Ingredients

- Water (10 cups)
- Cucumber (1 large, chopped)
- Celery (1 ½ Stalks quartered)
- Apples (2 large, seeded, quartered)
- Kale Leaves (2 Cups)
- Ginger (1-inch piece, peeled)

Directions
1. In a pitcher, combine all the ingredients.
2. Stir gently and refrigerate for at least 3 hours.
3. Serve after.

Macros per Serving & Nutrition Facts
- Calories 90.3
- Total Fat 0.0 g
- Carbohydrate 0.4 g

# Carrot and Papaya Coconut Water

This is very effective for eyes health and immune system.

Makes: 64 Fl.oz.
Time: 5 minutes + chilling time

Ingredients
- 2 carrots, peeled, sliced
- 1 cup ripe papaya, chunks
- 10 cups coconut water

Directions
1. Combine all ingredients in a pitcher.
2. Cover and allow to chill for a minimum of 2 hours or overnight.
3. Serve after.

Macros per Serving & Nutrition Facts
- Calories 93
- Total Fat 0.4 g
- Carbohydrate 22 g
- Protein 2.2g


## *Orange, Strawberry & Mint Infused Water*

If you frequently drink Mojitos, you will quickly find that replacing some of them with this mix will do wonders for your health.

Makes: 48fl. oz.
Time: 5 minutes + chilling time

Ingredients:
- 2 oranges, cut into wedges
- ½ cup strawberries
- 4 leaves mint
- 6 cups water

Directions
1. Place all the ingredients into a pitcher.
2. Cover and allow to chill for a minimum of 2 hours or overnight.
3. Serve after.

Macros per Serving & Nutrition Facts
- Calories 1.3
- Total Fat 0.0 g
- Carbohydrate 0.4 g
- Protein 0.0 g

# Watermelon Infused Coconut Water

This mix is said to aid in cardiovascular health as well as rejuvenating the skin.

Makes: 32 fl.oz.
Time: 5 minutes + chilling time

Ingredients:
- 4 cups coconut water
- 4 cups watermelon
- 2 tablespoons lime juice

Directions
1. Place all ingredients in a large pitcher,
2. Muddle gently and refrigerate for 2 hours.
3. Serve after, with some ice.

Macros per Serving & Nutrition Facts
- Calories 1.3
- Total Fat 0.0 g
- Carbohydrate 0.4 g
- Protein 0.0 g

# Raspberry, Kiwi & Peach Infused Water

This mix is perfect for flushing our bodies of unwanted toxins.

Makes: 64 fl. oz.
Time: 5 minutes + chilling time

Ingredients:
- 6 cups water
- 2 cups peaches, sliced
- 1 cup kiwi, sliced
- ½ cup raspberry

Directions
1. Combine all the ingredients in a pitcher.
2. Refrigerate for 2 hours or overnight.
3. Serve chilled!

Macros per Serving & Nutrition Facts
- Calories 1.3
- Total Fat 0.0 g
- Carbohydrate 0.4 g
- Protein 0.0 g

## *Peach & Sage Infused Water*

This mix is said to provide your body with some of the required antioxidants that will help your body fight bacteria and improve your overall health.

Makes: 64 fl. oz.
Time: 5 minutes + chilling time

Ingredients:
- 1 peach, pitted and sliced
- 8 pitted and quartered plums
- 4 sage leaves, scrunched
- 8 cups water

Directions
1. In a pitcher combine all the ingredients.
2. Give it a gentle stir and refrigerate at least 2 hours.
3. Serve with ice.

Macros per Serving & Nutrition Facts
- Calories 1.3
- Total Fat 0.0 g
- Carbohydrate 0.4 g
- Protein 0.0 g

# Kale & Apple Water

Though it may sound weird, this interesting blend creates a delicious and healthy juice.

Yields: 3 ½ Cups
Time Needed: 15 minutes

Ingredients
- Water (10 cups)
- Apples (4 large, seeded, quartered)
- Kale Leaves (3 Cups)
- Ginger (1-inch piece, peeled)

Directions
1. Place all the ingredients into a pitcher.
2. Cover and allow to chill for a minimum of 2 hours or overnight.
3. Serve after.

Macros per Serving & Nutrition Facts
- Calories 198
- Total Fat 3 g
- Carbohydrate 53 g
- Protein 19 g

# Watermelon & Mint Infused Water

Keep your body hydrated with this refreshing cup of water.

Makes: 64 fl. oz.
Time: 5 minutes + chilling time

Ingredients:
- 2 cups diced watermelon
- 4 mint leaves

- 10 cups water

Directions
1. In a pitcher combine the grapes and oranges.
2. Muddle gently and pour in the water.
3. Refrigerate for 2 hours.
4. Serve with ice.

Macros per Serving & Nutrition Facts
- Calories 1.3
- Total Fat 0.0 g
- Carbohydrate 0.4 g
- Protein 0.0 g

## _Orange & Grape Infused Water_

This mix is extremely tasty, offering a tangy, sweet, and refreshing mix.

Makes: 48 fl. oz.
Time: 5 minutes + chilling time

Ingredients:
- 1 cup halved red grapes, seedless
- 2 blood oranges, sliced
- 6 cups water

Directions
1. In a pitcher combine the grapes and oranges.
2. Muddle gently and pour in the water.
3. Refrigerate for 2 hours.
4. Serve with ice.

Macros per Serving & Nutrition Facts
- Calories 1.3
- Total Fat 0.0 g
- Carbohydrate 0.4 g
- Protein 0.0 g

## *Apple & Cinnamon Infused Water*

This delicious water blend is said to boost your metabolism naturally.

Makes: 64 fl. Oz.
Time: 5 minutes + chilling time

Ingredients:
- 2 apples, thinly sliced
- 1 cinnamon stick, preferably Ceylon cinnamon
- 8 cups water
- ½ jug of ice

Directions
1. Drop the apples in the pitcher and add the cinnamon stick.
2. Fill up with the ice up to ½ way full.
3. Top off with water and refrigerate for 1 hour.
4. Serve chilled.

Macros per Serving & Nutrition Facts
- Calories 1.3
- Total Fat 0.0 g
- Carbohydrate 0.4 g
- Protein 0.0 g

# Cherry Pineapple Infused Water

Use this mix to replace the sweet juices in your diet and watch in awe as the body starts to change before your eyes.

Makes: 64fl. oz.
Time: 5 minutes + chilling time

Ingredients:
- 1 cup pitted and halved cherries
- 1 cup pineapple chunks
- ½ green apple, cored and sliced
- 8 cups water

Directions
1. In a pitcher, combine all the ingredients.
2. Stir gently and refrigerate for at least 3 hours.
3. Serve after.

Macros per Serving & Nutrition Facts
- Calories 1.3
- Total Fat 0.0 g
- Carbohydrate 0.4 g
- Protein 0.0 g

# Ginger Zest Beetroot Water

This glass of infused water will make your skin and hair more glowing and shinier.

Makes: 48 fl. oz.
Time: 5 minutes + chilling time

Ingredients:
- 1 cup beetroots, peeled, chunks
- 1-inch ginger sliced, peeled

- 10 cups water

Directions
1. Place all ingredients in a large pitcher,
2. Muddle gently and refrigerate for 2 hours.
3. Serve after, with some ice.

Macros per Serving & Nutrition Facts
- Calories 155
- Total Fat 1 g
- Carbohydrate 33g
- Protein 1g

# *Kiwi & Blackberry Infused Water*

This mix is perfect for early mornings as it helps to set your metabolism in gear for the day ahead.

Makes: 32 fl. oz.
Time: 5 minutes + chilling time

Ingredients:
- ½ cup blackberries washed
- 1 kiwi, peeled and sliced
- 2 mint leaves
- 4 cups water

Directions
1. In a pitcher, combine all the ingredients.
2. Give it a gentle stir and refrigerate for 2 hours.
3. Serve after, with some ice.

Macros per Serving & Nutrition Facts
- Calories 1.3
- Total Fat 0.0 g
- Carbohydrate 0.4 g
- Protein 0.0 g

# _Broth Recipes_

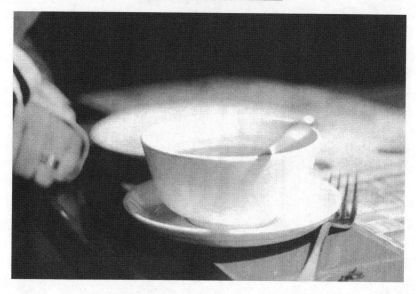

# Chicken Bone Broth

This recipe is perfect for soothing stomach aches

Preparation time: 2 hours
Yield: 5 servings

Ingredients
- 1 oz. chicken bones, cleaned
- 2 tablespoons apple cider vinegar
- 1 onion, sliced
- 5-6 garlic cloves
- 1 tablespoon cooking oil
- ½ teaspoon salt
- ½ teaspoon white pepper
- 1-inch ginger slice
- cups water

Directions
1. In a large skillet add bones with water, onion, garlic, ginger, oil, vinegar, salt, pepper, and stir. Cover with lid.
2. Leave to cook on low heat for 2 hours.
3. Strain the broth and discard residue.
4. Serve hot and enjoy.

Macros per Serving & Nutrition Facts
- Calories 147
- Total Fat 5 g
- Carbohydrate 9 g
- Protein 10 g

# _Pork Bone Broth_

This highly nutritious delight is made with just a few and simple ingredients.

Preparation time: 2 hours
Yield: 5 servings

Ingredients
- 1 oz. pork bones, cleaned
- 2 tablespoons apple cider vinegar
- 1 onion, sliced
- 5-6 garlic cloves
- 1 tablespoon cooking oil
- ½ teaspoon salt
- ½ teaspoon white pepper
- 1-inch ginger slice
- cups water

Directions
1. In a large skillet add bones with water, onion, garlic, ginger, oil, vinegar, salt, pepper, and stir. Cover with lid.
2. Leave to cook on low heat for 2 hours.
3. Strain the broth and discard residue.
4. Serve hot and enjoy.

Macros per Serving & Nutrition Facts
- Calories 37.7
- Total Fat 0.2 g
- Carbohydrate 8.2 g
- Protein 1 g

# Conclusion

There you have it! Together we have explored 50 Amazingly Simple Recipes that you can enjoy within Stage 1 of recovery from a Gastric Sleeve Operation. We hope you will consider joining us again when we explore the remaining three stages of post operation diet procedures. Achieving a speedy and successful recovery is vital right now, and we want to help you get there. See you next time.

# *Gastric Sleeve Cookbook Stage 2*

50 Delicious Protein Shakes & Smoothies, Soups and Puddings Recipes You Can Enjoy in Stage 2 Post Weight Loss Surgery Rehabilitation

**Copyright © 2018 Victoria Goode**

**All Rights Reserved.**

**Disclaimer Notice**

The following is intended for informational purposes only. Patients take all responsibility and must consult their doctor.

# Table of Contents

# Introduction

Congratulations, once again, on successfully completing your gastric sleeve surgery and making it successfully into your second stage of the recovery diet! So, stage 1 consuming only clear fluids was a success, and you are ready to move on to stage 2 which primarily has thicker liquids and slowly introducing smooth foods into the diet. Before you proceed to this stage it is important that you check your fluid consumption log and ask yourself if you can comfortably consume a suitable amount of liquid daily without experiencing added pouch irritation, discomfort, and vomiting? If so, then great; feel free to move on to stage 2 confidently. However, if you are still not quite there, don't rush yourself. Instead, consider sticking to stage 1 for a few more days to a week until you are able to comfortably move on. Remember, every patient is different so your body may heal differently than others. Listen to your body, and adjust your recovery process to suit your body and specific needs.

## _So, what should you expect to achieve in Stage 2?_

In this stage of your diet you will be introducing more full liquids to your diet, so when you are just transitioning from stage 1, you will start to try your body with digesting more shakes, milk, skimmed milk, sugar free soft puddings, and maybe even sugar free porridges. In this stage, you want to aim to consume at least 6 to 8 fluid ounces of liquid per hour while taking more frequent smaller portions of food. Then towards the end of the stage when you begin to transition to stage 3 then you will start testing yourself with the introduction of soft or smooth foods in an attempt to get your body prepared for stage 3. Don't be scared! You can definitely get through this. Just ensure that you keep these few key tips in mind as you go through this stage.

## _Stage 2 Key Tips/Reminders_

- In this stage protein shakes will be your best friend. Meeting your nutritional targets daily as the stages go by will become more and more vital to a tall glass of a protein shake will help you along with meeting those pesky protein targets.

- When you get into the second week of this stage when you begin to introduce smooth foods to your diet, be sure that you do not force yourself to eat. Listen to your body! If you do not feel really hungry, opt to try drinking a small glass of protein shake versus a whole serving of your scheduled smooth meal.

- Be sure that you pace yourself while you eat. Try to take dime sized bites and allow your body to process that before jumping to binge on more.

- When you begin to try smooth foods, aim to have your food the consistency of apple sauce so that it can be easily digested without too much discomfort. Even if your food appears to be smooth always chew thoroughly before attempting to swallow.

- It is important to stay hydrated! Try to continue t sip on clear fluids in between meals. Try not to drink too much close to your schedule meal times as you want to leave space in your stomach for the actual meal. Remember your stomach is not able to hold as much as it could before so over eating may result in vomiting or discomfort.

- Keep a log of the nutrients you are consuming and be sure to supplement the nutrients you fall short on (many patients fall short on their protein, B12, and Calcium intake during the first couple of stages so check with your doctor if taking a pill is necessary in your case).

- Try to eat at set times throughout the day and stick to it. That way you can ensure you are actually consuming enough food for your body. Try to eat at least every 4 hours while you are awake.

- Aim to consume at least 64 fluid ounces of liquid each day. This may sound like a lot, however, remember that there is liquid in your shakes so track that first then supplement your fluid intake with clear liquids throughout the day.

This is a lot of information to take in, but it really isn't as complicated as it sounds. In this Gastric Sleeve Cookbook, we are going to help keep you on track with 50 Delicious recipe suggestions that you can enjoy in Stage 2 of your post gastric sleeve recovery diet. We guarantee that once you see how simple it can be things will begin to become clearer. So, without further ado, let's get started.

# Introducing Full Liquids

## _Protein Shakes & Smoothies_

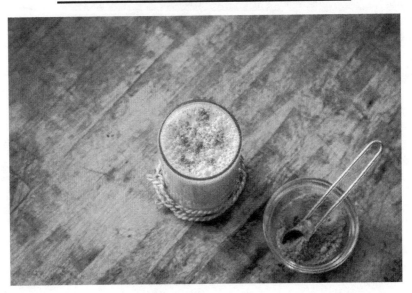

# Pineapple Shake V 20

This sweet and tasty drink is a brilliant end to a heavy meal.

Serves: 6
Time: 20 minutes

Ingredients:
- Frozen pineapple (3 cups)
- Whey Protein Powder (2 scoops)
- Greek yogurt (1 cup, pineapple/vanilla flavored)
- Unsweetened vanilla almond milk (1 cup)
- Vanilla extract (1 tbs.)

Directions:
1. Add the ingredients in the blender and blend until smooth.
2. Serve and enjoy!

Macros per Serving & Nutrition Facts
- Calories 580
- Total Fat 31 g
- Total Carbohydrate 68 g
- Protein 28g

# Blueberry Cacao Blast V 20

Simple yet delicious dessert smoothie.

Serves: 1
Time: 5 minutes

Ingredients:
- 1 cup blueberries
- 1 tablespoon raw cacao nibs
- 1 tablespoon Chia seeds
- 1 dash cinnamon

- ½ Spinach (chopped)
- ½ Cup Bananas (chopped)
- 1½ Cup Almond milk
- 2 scoops Whey protein powder

Directions:
1. Place raspberries, cacao nibs, Chia seeds and cinnamon in a blender.
2. Add enough almond milk to reach the max line.
3. Process for 30 seconds or until you get a smooth mixture.
4. Serve immediately in the chilled tall glass.

Macros per Serving & Nutrition Facts
- Calories 321
- Total Fat 2.7 g
- Total Carbohydrate 69.4 g
- Protein 24.7g

## *Cucumber and Avocado Dill Smoothie V 20*

If you are looking for a delicious and healthy smoothie, then this is perfect for you.

Serves: 2
Time: 5 minutes

Ingredients:
- 1 cucumber, peeled, sliced
- 2 tablespoons dill, chopped
- 2 tablespoons lemon juice
- 1 avocado, pitted
- 1 cup coconut milk
- 1 teaspoon coconut, shredded
- 2 kiwis, peeled, sliced

Directions
1. In a blender add all ingredients and blend well.
2. Drain the extract and discard residue.
3. Serve and enjoy.

Macros per Serving & Nutrition Facts
- Calories 165
- Total Fat 5.5 g
- Total Carbohydrate 24.8 g
- Protein 2.3g

## *Spinach Green Smoothie V 20*

This smoothie will definitely blow your mind by its taste and freshness.

Serves: 2
Time: 5 min

Ingredients:
- 1 cup baby spinach leaves
- 2-3 mint leave
- 1 cup 100% grapes juice
- 1 cup 100% pineapple juice
- 2 tablespoons lime juice
- 2 scoops protein powder

Directions
1. In a blender add ingredients and blend well till puree.
2. Transfer to serving glasses.
3. Serve and enjoy.

Macros per Serving & Nutrition Facts
- Calories 268
- Total Fat 5.5 g
- Total Carbohydrate 11.4 g
- Protein 24.3g

# Coco - Banana Milkshake V 20

Here is a delicious milkshake that is naturally sweet from the coconut and bananas.

Serves: 1
Time: 5 minutes

Ingredients
- 1 cup coconut milk
- 2 ripe bananas
- 2 tablespoons cinnamon
- ¼ teaspoon cardamom powder
- 2 scoops protein powder
- 7 ice cubes

Directions
1. In a blender add coconut milk with cardamom powder, cinnamon, bananas and blend well.
2. Pour into glass and add ice chunks.
3. Serve and enjoy.

Macros per Serving & Nutrition Facts
- Calories 191.9
- Total Fat 7.1g
- Total Carbohydrate 35.8 g
- Protein 25.7g

# Strawberry and Cherry Shake V 20

This shake is absolutely a great boost with wonderful taste.

Serves:2
Time: 5 minutes

Ingredients:

- 1 cup strawberries
- 1 cup cherries
- 1 cup almond milk
- ½ cup coconut milk
- 2 scoops protein powder
- Few ice chunks

Directions
1. In a blender add all ingredients and blend well.
2. Serve and enjoy.

Macros per Serving & Nutrition Facts
- Calories 138
- Total Fat 0g
- Total Carbohydrate 30 g
- Protein 20g

## Chia Blueberry Banana Oatmeal Smoothie V 20

Banana check, blueberry check, starting the day right, check.

Serves: 1
Time: 10m

Ingredients:
- Soy milk (1 cups)
- Frozen banana (1, sliced)
- Frozen blueberries (1/4 cup)
- Oats (1/4 cup)
- Vanilla extract (1 tsp.)
- Cinnamon (1 tsp., to taste)
- Chia seed (1 tbs.)

Directions:
1. Add all ingredients into a blender and blend until the ingredients are combined and smooth.

2. Serve and enjoy!

Macros per Serving & Nutrition Facts
- Calories 178
- Total Fat 4.2 g
- Total Carbohydrate 36.2 g
- Protein 3.2 g

# *Chocolate Coconut Chia Smoothie V 20*

This smoothie is packed with protein and filled with sweet chocolaty flavor.

Serves: 1
Time: 5 minutes

Ingredients:
- 1 tablespoon raw cacao nibs
- 1 tablespoon Chia seeds
- 1 dash cinnamon
- ½ Spinach (chopped)
- ½ Cup Coconut (shredded)
- 1½ Cup Almond milk

Directions:
1. Place coconut, cacao nibs, Chia seeds and cinnamon in Vitamix.
2. Add enough almond milk to reach the max line.
3. Process for 30 seconds or until you get a smooth mixture.
4. Serve immediately in the tall chilled glass.

Macros per Serving & Nutrition Facts
- Calories 480
- Total Fat 22 g
- Total Carbohydrate 55 g
- Protein 30 g

# Banana-Cherry Smoothie V 20

Cherries are great in combatting inflammation in the body and

Serves: 1
Time: 5 minutes

Ingredients:
- 1 banana
- 1 cup cherries, pitted
- ¼ teaspoon nutmeg
- 1scoop protein powder
- 1 cup almond milk

Directions:
1. Place all ingredients in a blender
2. Process ingredients until smooth, for 20 seconds.
3. Serve immediately.

Macros per Serving & Nutrition Facts
- Calories 398
- Total Fat 2 g
- Total Carbohydrate 89.2 g
- Protein 17 g

# Avocado Smoothie V 20

This recipe produces a creamy and delicious green smoothie providing a healthy source of fat.

Serves: 1
Time: 5 minutes

Ingredients:
- 1 medium ripe avocado
- ¼ cup crushed peanuts
- 1 tablespoon flax seed
- 1 ½ cups vanilla Greek yogurt
- 1 cup Liquid (milk, water, coconut milk, etc.)

Directions:
1. Place all ingredients in Vitamix.
2. Process ingredients until smooth, for 20 seconds.
3. Serve immediately.

Macros per Serving & Nutrition Facts
- Calories 592
- Total Fat 22 g
- Total Carbohydrate 96 g
- Protein 3 g

# *Mango Smoothie V 20*

Enjoy this rich tropical mango smoothie that will remind you of the islands.

Serves: 2
Time: 5 minutes

Ingredients:
- 2 Mangos (seeded, diced, frozen)
- Milk (1 cup)
- ½ cup crushed ice
- 1 cup plain yogurt
- 2 scoops protein powder

Directions:
1. Combine all ingredients in Vitamix.
2. Process for 30 seconds or until smooth.
3. Serve immediately in a tall glass.

Macros per Serving & Nutrition Facts
- Calories 320
- Total Fat 0 g
- Total Carbohydrate 78 g
- Protein 21 g

# *Homemade Unsweetened Milk*

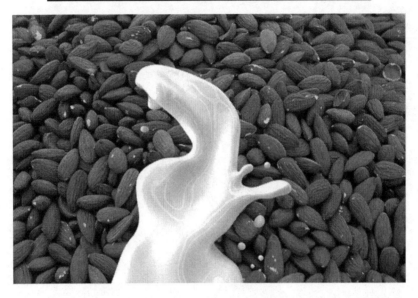

# Cashew Milk V 20

Who says you have to pay a fortune for Cashew Milk? Get fresh homemade cashew milk using your Vitamix right from your kitchen.

Serves: 5
Time:15min.

Ingredients
- Cashew (1 Cup. Soaked over time)
- Water (4 cups)
- Dates (3)

DIRECTIONS
1. Add all your ingredients to your Vitamix.
2. Pulse for until creamy (should take about 1 min).
3. Enjoy!

Macros per Serving & Nutrition Facts
- Calories 60
- Total Fat 2.5 g
- Total Carbohydrate 27.3 g
- Protein 8 g

# Almond Milk V 20

Almond milk does not have to be expensive. Using this recipe, you can enjoy fresh Almond Milk from your kitchen.

Serves: 5 cups
Time Needed: 15min.

Ingredients
- Almonds (1 Cup. Soaked over time)
- Water (4 cups)

Directions

1. Add all your ingredients to your Vitamix.
2. Pulse for until creamy (should take about 1 min).
3. Enjoy!

Macros per Serving & Nutrition Facts

- Calories 90
- Total Fat 2.5 g
- Total Carbohydrate 16 g
- Protein 1 g

# Strained Soups

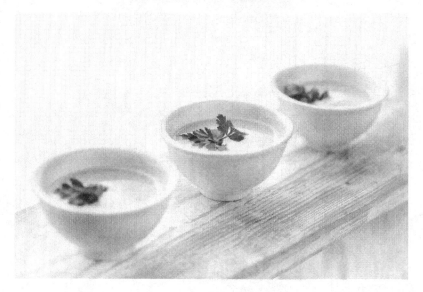

# *Pumpkin and carrot soup V 20*

Super healthy and vibrant soup everyone will love.

Serves: 4
Time: 20 minutes

Ingredients:
- 0.5 lb. pumpkin puree
- 0.5 lb. carrots, cut into ½-inch pieces
- 2 cups vegetable stock
- ½ cup chopped onion
- Fresh ground salt and pepper – to taste
- 1 teaspoon dried thyme
- 2 oz. cauliflower florets
- ½ tablespoon olive oil
- 1 anise star

Direction:
1. Heat olive oil in medium pot and add onion; add cauliflower, carrots and sauté for 15 minutes, until onion is caramelized.
2. Add thyme and stir well.
3. Transfer the vegetables in a Nutri Bullet, add pumpkin puree, vegetable stock, and pulse until smooth.
4. Transfer the mixture into sauce pan and simmer, add anise star and simmer over medium-high heat for 5-8 minutes or until heated through.
5. Remove the anise star and discard.
6. Strain through a fine sieve or cheesecloth and serve immediately.

Macros per Serving & Nutrition Facts
- Calories 70
- Total Fat 0 g
- Total Carbohydrate 0 g
- Protein 2 g

# _Super Soup_

Why Super soup? Well, it is packed with the super ingredients and has a super taste.

Serves: 6
Time: 30 minutes

Ingredients:
- 14oz. cauliflower heat, cut into florets
- 5oz. watercress
- 7oz. spinach, thawed
- cups chicken stock
- 1 cup coconut milk
- ¼ cup ghee
- Salt and pepper – to taste
- 1 onion, chopped
- 2 garlic cloves, crushed

Directions:
1. Grease Dutch oven with ghee, place over medium-high heat and add onion and garlic. Cook until browned and stir cauliflower florets. Cook for 5 minutes.
2. Add spinach and water cress and cook for 2 minutes or until just wilted, pour in vegetable stock and bring to boil.
3. Cook until cauliflower is crisp-tender and stir in the coconut milk.
4. Season with salt and pepper and remove from the heat. Allow cooling and puree the soup in Nutri Bullet until creamy.
5. Strain through a fine sieve or cheesecloth and serve immediately.

Macros per Serving & Nutrition Facts
- Calories 392
- Total Fat 37.6 g

- Total Carbohydrate 9.7 g
- Protein 4.9 g

# *Tomato bisque*

This soup has a kind of pizza aroma. It is filled with tomatoes and basil.

Serves: 4
Time: 30 minutes

Ingredients:
- 28oz. tomatoes, peeled and pureed
- 1 cup coconut cream
- 1 onion, diced
- 1 teaspoon fresh ground pepper
- cups chicken stock
- 1 bunch celery, chopped
- ½ cup basil, chopped
- 1 tablespoon olive oil
- Salt and pepper – to taste

Directions:
1. Heat olive oil in large pot over medium-high heat, add onion, with celery and cook until tender.
2. Pour chicken stock and tomatoes in the pot, bring mixture to simmer and season with salt and pepper. Simmer for 30 minutes.
3. Turn off heat and allow the soup to cool down. Puree in Nutri Bullet in batches.
4. Stir in heavy cream, basil, and Parmesan cheese.
5. Strain through a fine sieve or cheesecloth and serve immediately.

Macros per Serving & Nutrition Facts
- Calories 140
- Total Fat 7 g
- Total Carbohydrate 17 g
- Protein 3 g

## *Smoky soup V*

Soup made with smoked paprika, bell peppers and with a pinch of ginger.

Serves: 4
Time: 40 minutes

Ingredients:
- 3 red bell peppers, diced
- 1 ½ tablespoons grass-fed butter
- 2 carrots, grated
- 1 brown onion, diced
- 2 garlic cloves, minced
- 1 ½ tablespoon tomato puree
- 2 teaspoons fresh grated ginger
- 1 teaspoon smoked paprika
- 1 bay leaf
- ½ cup chilled coconut cream whisked with 1 tablespoon lemon juice
- cups homemade vegetable stock
- ½ teaspoon ground coriander

Directions:
1. Melt butter in medium heavy-bottom pan, over medium-high heat.
2. Add carrots, bell peppers, and onion. Cook for 13-15 minutes or until onion is golden, stirring occasionally.
3. Add garlic, ginger, smoked paprika, tomato puree and coriander.

4   Cook until very fragrant, for 2 minutes.
5   Add bay leaf and stock; bring to boil and reduce heat to medium-low and simmer for 20-25 minutes.
6   Remove bay leaf and when cooled puree in batches using Nutribullet. Process until smooth.
7   Stir Strain in a fine sieve or cheesecloth and serve immediately.

Macros per Serving & Nutrition Facts
- Calories 100
- Total Fat 2 g
- Total Carbohydrate 16 g
- Protein 5 g

# *Chicken Ramen Soup Broth*

If you love ramen, you will love this recipe. It uses chicken instead of pork for all the chicken lovers.

Serves: 2-3
Time: 1 hr.

Ingredients:
- Onion, large, diced (1)
- Carrots, diced (2)
- Celery, diced (3)
- Garlic, finely chopped (4 cloves)
- Kosher salt (1 tsp)
- Pepper (½ tsp)
- Cinnamon (2 tsp)
- Chicken broth, low sodium (6)
- Light Miso (2 tsp)
- Chicken breasts (1 lb.)
- Spinach (1 bag)

Directions

1. Prepare carrots, celery, and onions for cooking in a latch Dutch oven for 5-7 minutes over medium heat. Now include salt, pepper, cinnamon, and garlic, and continue to cook for an additional minute.
2. Add chicken broth and miso before bringing to a boil.
3. Now add whole chicken breasts (raw), and simmer. Continue for 10-12 minutes. Occasionally remove a chicken breast and cut it, to see if it is cooked.
4. When the chicken is cooked thoroughly, relocate it to a cutting board for cooling.
5. When the chicken is cool enough to be handled, mince it finely, then add it back into the vegetable broth.
6. Stir in spinach to cook for approximately 5 minutes until spinach is tender.
7. Serve and enjoy!

Macros per Serving & Nutrition Facts
- Calories 326.9
- Total Fat 13.4 g
- Total Carbohydrate 39.7 g
- Protein 10.3 g

## *Carrot, Ginger Gusto Apple Soup*

You will be surprised with this yummy soup.

Serves: 3
Preparation time: 35 minutes

Ingredients:
- 2 cup yellow apple, chunks, peeled
- 1 cup boiled chicken, shredded
- 1 carrot, peeled and chopped
- ¼ cup cherries, chopped

- 2 cups chicken broth
- 1 tablespoons lemon juice
- 1 teaspoon ginger paste
- ½ teaspoon black pepper
- ¼ teaspoon salt
- 1 tablespoon oil

Directions
1. Heat oil in a pan, add ginger paste and fry for 1 minute.
2. Add all chicken and carrots, then fry well.
3. Season with salt and pepper.
4. Transfer apple chunks, strawberries, chicken broth and stir well.
5. Place to cook on low fire for 30 minutes.
6. Drizzle lemon juice.
7. Strain, and ladle into serving bowls.
8. Serve and enjoy.

Macros per Serving & Nutrition Facts
- Calories 172.3
- Total Fat 8.7 g
- Total Carbohydrate 22.7 g
- Protein 3.2 g

## *Carrot, Ginger Zest Chicken Orangey Soup 20*

This soup is the combination of orange slices and chicken with the flavor of ginger.

Serves: 3
Time: 15 minutes

Ingredients:
- 1 oz. chicken bones or boiled chicken feet
- 2 oranges, sliced, seeded

- carrots, peeled and chopped
- 2 cups chicken broth
- 1 teaspoon ginger paste
- ½ teaspoon chili powder
- ¼ teaspoon salt
- 1 tablespoon oil

Directions
1. Heat oil in a pan, add ginger paste and carrot, then cook for 1 minute.
2. Add chicken, salt, chili powder and fry till golden brown.
3. Add chicken broth, orange slice and stir.
4. Leave to cook on low heat for 15 minutes.
5. Strain and ladle into serving bowls.
6. Serve and enjoy.

Macros per Serving & Nutrition Facts
- Calories 159
- Total Fat 3 g
- Total Carbohydrate 27 g
- Protein 6 g

## *Rice Cooker Garden soup*

Enjoy delicious soup made of different veggies and chewy bulgur.

Serves: 6
Time: 50 minutes

Ingredients:
- 15oz. can chickpeas, rinsed and drained
- 2 carrots, diced
- 2 zucchinis, trimmed, cubed
- 2 sprigs thyme
- 1 leek, white and light green parts chopped
- ½ cup bulgur

- 4oz. green beans, cut into ½-inch pieces
- cups water
- 2 garlic cloves, minced
- 2 cups chicken stock
- tablespoons butter
- 1 cup tomatoes, chopped
- 1 cup fresh peas
- 1 bay leaf
- Salt and pepper, to taste

Directions:
1. Set your rice cooker to white rice.
2. Add the butter and once melted add the celery, chickpeas, leek, garlic, zucchinis, garlic.
3. Cook, stirring for 4 minutes.
4. Add the stock, bulgur, tomatoes, bay leaf, water, and thyme.
5. Simmer for 30 minutes. Add the green beans and peas. Discard the thyme. Cook for 5 minutes.
6. Serve after.

Macros per Serving & Nutrition Facts
- Calories 100
- Total Fat 3.5 g
- Total Carbohydrate 18 g
- Protein 3 g

## Lemony Chicken Soup Broth

A zest of fresh lemon juice infuses this tasty Chicken soup. Other rich spices help to make the experience fun!

Serves: 2-3
Time: 1 hr.
Ingredients
- Onion, large, diced (1)

- Carrots, diced (2)
- Celery, diced (3)
- Garlic, finely chopped (4 cloves)
- Kosher salt (1 tsp)
- Pepper (½ tsp)
- Cinnamon (2 tsp)
- Chicken broth, low sodium (6)
- Parsley, extra for garnish (10 sprigs)
- Chicken breasts (1 lb.)
- Spinach (1 bag)
- Chick peas, canned, washed/drained (15 ounces)
- Juice of a Lemon (½ lemon, or more to taste)

Directions

1. Prepare carrots, celery, and onions for cooking in a latch Dutch oven for 5-7 minutes over medium heat. Now include salt, pepper, cinnamon, and garlic, and continue to cook for an additional minute.
2. Add whole parsley sprigs to your pot and stir in chicken broth before bringing to a boil.
3. Now add whole chicken breasts (raw), and simmer. Continue for 10-12 minutes. Occasionally remove a chicken breast and cut it, to see if it is cooked.
4. When the chicken is cooked thoroughly, relocate it to a cutting board for cooling.
5. When the chicken is cool enough to be handled, shred it, then add it back into the vegetable broth.
6. Stir in lemon juice, chick peas, and spinach to cook for approximately 5 minutes until spinach is tender.
7. Strain the soup to gather the broth and discard the solids, garnish with newly chopped parsley, and enjoy!

Macros per Serving & Nutrition Facts
- Calories 252.8
- Total Fat 8 g
- Total Carbohydrate 19.8 g
- Protein 25.6 g

# Introducing Smooth & Pureed Foods

## *Sugar Free Puddings & Treats*

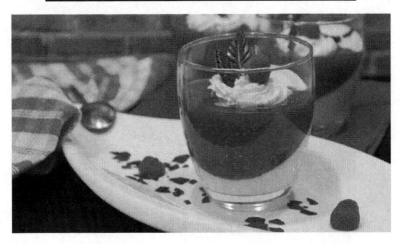

# *Chocolate and Banana Pudding V*

Make this pudding and place in the fridge for better results.

Serves: 5
Preparation time: 2 hours

Ingredients
- 1 cup almond milk
- 1 cup chocolate, melted
- bananas, peeled, sliced
- ½ cup condensed almond milk
- 2 tablespoons butter
- 2 tablespoons cocoa powder
- 1 cup coconut cream

Directions
1. In a sauce pan add butter with and leave to cook until reduced to half.
2. Now add condensed almond milk, chocolate, cocoa powder, and stir gradually.
3. Pour half of chocolate pudding into a large dish and place banana slices evenly.
4. Pour remaining chocolate on top and freeze for 2 hours.
5. Top with whipped cream before serving.
6. Enjoy.

Macros per Serving & Nutrition Facts

- Calories 187.3
- Total Fat 3.6 g
- Total Carbohydrate 34.7 g
- Protein 4.4 g

# *Pomegranate Pudding V*

This recipe is sugar free, and it has pomegranate for added sweetness

Serves: 4
Time: 4 hours and 35 minutes

Ingredients:
- Pomegranate juice (1 cup)
- Pomegranate juice (1/4 cup)
- Agar Agar flakes (1 tbs.)
- Tapioca starch (1 tsp.)
- Protein Powder (1 scoop)

Directions:
1. In a saucepan add the 1 cup of pomegranate juice and the agar agar. On medium heat bring it to a simmer and stir occasionally. Once the pot starts to simmer, lower the temperature to a lower heat for a 1 minute.
2. In a cup add the ¼ cup of the remaining pomegranate juice and the tapioca. Stir well. Add this mixture to the sauce pan and stir well.
3. Pour the mixture into a serving cup and put it in the fridge for 4 hours so that the Jell-O set.
4. Serve and enjoy!

Macros per Serving & Nutrition Facts
- Calories 57
- Total Fat 0 g
- Total Carbohydrate 12 g
- Protein 12 g

# *Carrot Pudding V*

Creamy carrot pudding with a delicate lemony aroma.

Serves: 6
Time: 30 minutes

Ingredients:
- 2/3 cup Carrot Puree
- 1 teaspoon vanilla paste
- 1 teaspoon lemon zest
- cups coconut milk
- Cornstarch Slurry (mixture of 2 tbs. cornstarch and 4tbs. water)
- 1 egg

Directions:
1. Place the carrot and milk into a saucepan over low heat.
2. Cover and cook until tiny bubbles begin to form.
3. Meanwhile, whisk the egg, cornstarch slurry, and lemon zest then add to the pot in a steady stream.
4. Cover and cook for 15 minutes.
5. Divide the mix between dessert bowls.
6. Cool before serving.

Macros per Serving & Nutrition Facts
- Calories 159
- Total Fat 10 g
- Total Carbohydrate 18 g
- Protein 4 g

## Yogurt Crème Brulee Custard V 20

Who says a yogurt can be served only in one way? We bring you something really special.

Serves: 4
Time: 5 minutes

Ingredients:
- 2 cup thick Greek yogurt
- 1 cup strawberries puree

Directions:
1. In a bowl, combine the strawberries puree with yogurt.
2. Divide the mix between four ramekins.
3. Serve after.

Macros per Serving & Nutrition Facts
- Calories 357.6
- Total Fat 27 g
- Total Carbohydrate 22.2 g
- Protein 5.9 g

## *Mango Chia Pudding V*

Now you can enjoy the taste of mango in the morning.

Serves: 6
Time: 2h 10m

Ingredients:
- Flax milk (1 ½ cups, coconut flavored)
- Large mango (1, cut into chunks)
- Vanilla extract (1 tsp.)
- Tea salt (1/8 tsp.)
- Chia seed (7 tbs.)
- Cinnamon (3 tbs.)

Directions:
1. Add all ingredients into a blender and blend until the ingredients are combined and smooth.
2. Put the mixture into a bowl and it in the fridge for 2 hours or until it thickens.

3. Serve and enjoy!

Macros per Serving & Nutrition Facts
- Calories 159
- Total Fat 10 g
- Total Carbohydrate 18 g
- Protein 4 g

# *Chocolate Mousse V 20*

Chocolate mousse prepared in a blender. Rich and decadent.

Serves: 2
Time: 5 minutes

Ingredients:
- ¼ cup unsweetened dark chocolate
- 1¾ cups heavy whipping cream
- ½ teaspoon orange extract
- ¼ Cup cinnamon
- ½ cup whip cream (to serve)
- ¼ cup dark unsweetened chocolate (shaved, to serve)

Directions:
1  Place all ingredients into a blender.
2  Process until desired consistency is reached.
3  Chill, and top with whip cream and shaved chocolate before serving.

Macros per Serving & Nutrition Facts
- Calories 40
- Total Fat 3 g
- Total Carbohydrate 3 g
- Protein 1 g

# Lemon Crème Brulee Custard V

Creamy, tasty and decadent without the super crunchy sugar crust.

Serves: 5
Time: 50 minutes + inactive time

Ingredients:
- egg yolks, whisked
- 1 tablespoons cinnamon
- ½ teaspoon lemon extract
- 1 teaspoon lemon zest
- ½ teaspoon vanilla extract
- 2 cups heavy coconut cream, chilled

Directions:
1. In a large heavy-bottom sauce pan, over medium heat, heat whipping cream cinnamon until bubbly around the sides of the pan.
2. Remove from the heat and add 1 tablespoon of heated cream into egg yolks; whisk well and pour the egg mixture into hot cream, stirring constantly.
3. Stir in the extracts and lemon zest, whisking well.
4. Preheat oven to 325F and pour the mixture into six 6 oz. ramekins.
5. Place ramekins into baking pan and pour around 1 cup water; set in the oven and bake uncovered for 30 minutes or until center is just set.
6. Remove ramekins from the hot bath and cook for 10 minutes.
7. Cover and refrigerate for 4 hours.
8. Serve immediately.

Macros per Serving & Nutrition Facts
- Calories 198
- Total Fat 15.7 g

- Total Carbohydrate 12.2 g
- Protein 2.6 g

# *Raisin and Oats Mug Cakes V 20*

Do you love oatmeal and want another way to make a creative dish with them? Why not make a mug cake?

Serves: 1
Time: 3 minutes

Ingredients
- Flour (1 ½ tbsp.)
- Almond milk (1 ½ tbsp.)
- Raisins (1/2 tbsp.)
- Baking powder (1/4 teaspoon)
- Salt (1/16 tsp. to taste)
- Canola oil (1/2 tbsp.)
- Baking soda (1/8 teaspoons)
- Vanilla extract (1/8 teaspoon)
- Hazelnut extract (1/8 teaspoon)
- Oats (3/4 tbsps., apple cinnamon)
- Lemon Juice (1 tsp.)

*Directions*
1  Whisk all ingredients in a microwavable mug and place to cook on high for a minute.
2  Cool, serve and enjoy!

Macros per Serving & Nutrition Facts
- Calories 185
- Total Fat 1.7 g
- Total Carbohydrate 39.9 g
- Protein 7.6 g

# _Thicker/Creamier Soups_

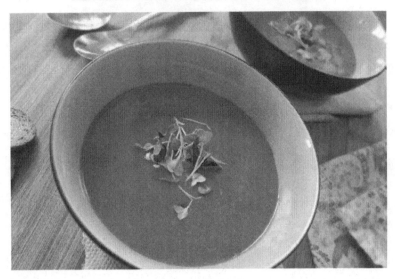

# *Onion and Peas Soup*

A simple and colorful soup that with blow your mind.

Serves: 3
Time: 25 minutes

Ingredients
- 1 cup peas, boiled
- carrots, peeled, chopped
- 1 onion, sliced
- 2 cups chicken broth
- 1 tablespoons lemon juice
- 4-5 garlic cloves, minced
- ½ teaspoon black pepper
- ¼ teaspoon salt
- 1 tablespoon oil

Directions
1 Heat oil in a saucepan, add onion and garlic cloves, fry for 2 minutes.
2 Add all peas and carrots stir for 5 minutes.
3 Add chicken broth, salt, pepper, and mix well.
4 Leave to cook on low heat for 15 minutes.
5 Strain and ladle into serving bowls.
6 Drizzle lemon juice.
7 Serve and enjoy.

Macros per Serving & Nutrition Facts
- Calories 115
- Total Fat 0 g
- Total Carbohydrate 21 g
- Protein 7 g

# *Curried Carrot, Sweet Potato, and Ginger Soup V*

Cholesterol isn't an issue when enjoying this delicious creamy soup, as it Is filled with Beta-Carotene and Vitamin A which together helps to promote healthy vision.

Serves: 3
Time: 30 – 35min

Ingredients:
- Extra Virgin Olive Oil (2 tsp.)
- Shallots (½ cup, chopped)
- Sweet Potato (3 cups, peeled, cubed)
- Carrots (1½ cup, peeled, sliced)

Directions:
1. Place a saucepan with your oil on medium heat until it just begins to smoke.
2. Add your shallots to the pot and sauté until it becomes tender (should take approximately 2 – 3 min).
3. Add all your prepped vegetables to the shallots, and your curry then allow to cook for another 2 minutes.
4. Pour in your broth and allow it to come to a boil. Once boiling, place the lid on the pot and reduce the heat to low.
5. Allow this mixture to simmer until your vegetables are all tender.
6. Once tender, add salt and pour your soup into a food processor. Pulse until creamy and smooth.
7. Strain, serve and Enjoy.

Tip: Consider topping with a teaspoon of vanilla Greek yogurt and sesame seeds.

Macros per Serving & Nutrition Facts
- Calories 144
- Total Fat 2.3 g
- Total Carbohydrate 27.3 g
- Protein 4.1 g

# *Creamy Cauliflower Soup*

Get a creamy cauliflower soup just like they do in the restaurants.

Serves: 6
Time: 30 minutes

Ingredients:
- 14oz. cauliflower heat, cut into florets
- 5oz. watercress
- 7oz. spinach, thawed
- cups chicken stock
- ¼ cup ghee
- Salt and pepper – 1 tsp. each to taste
- 1 onion, chopped
- garlic cloves, crushed

Directions:
1. Grease Dutch oven with ghee, place over medium-high heat and add onion and garlic. Cook until browned and stir cauliflower florets. Cook for 5 minutes.
2. Add spinach and water cress and cook for 2 minutes or until just wilted, pour in vegetable stock and bring to boil.
3. Cook until cauliflower is crisp-tender and stir in the coconut milk.
4. Season with salt and pepper and remove from the heat. Allow cooling and puree the soup in Vitamix until creamy.
5. Strain and serve immediately.

Macros per Serving & Nutrition Facts
- Calories 105
- Total Fat 8 g
- Total Carbohydrate 6 g
- Protein 4 g

# *Cream of Corn Soup V*

This classic and delicious treat can become even more smooth when finished in a Vitamix.

Serves: 4
Time Needed: 25 minutes

Ingredients:
- 0.5 lb. Corn puree
- 0.5 lb. carrots, cut into ½-inch pieces
- cups vegetable stock
- ½ cup chopped onion
- ½ teaspoon Salt
- ¼ teaspoon Pepper
- 1 teaspoon dried thyme
- oz. celery (chopped)
- ½ tablespoon olive oil
- 1 anise star

Directions:
1. Heat olive oil in medium pot and add onion; add celery, carrots and sauté for 15 minutes, until onion is caramelized. Add in corn and stir until corn is tender.
2. Add thyme and stir well.
3. Transfer the vegetables in a Vitamix, add pumpkin puree, vegetable stock, and pulse until smooth.
4. Transfer the mixture into sauce pan and simmer, add anise star and simmer over medium-high heat for 5-8 minutes or until heated through.
5. Remove the anise star and discard.
6. Serve immediately.

Macros per Serving & Nutrition Facts
- Calories 294
- Total Fat 8.3 g
- Total Carbohydrate 56 g
- Protein 12.9 g

# *Chestnut Soup*

The soup is a combination of heavy cream, roasted chestnuts, and bacon. The perfect soup for the perfect autumn day.

Serves: 6
Time: 45 minutes

Ingredients:
- 30oz. whole roasted chestnuts
- 1 shallot, roughly chopped
- bacon slices, chopped
- ½ cup heavy cream
- ½ cups chicken stock
- 1 leek, white and light green parts chopped
- tablespoons butter
- 1 sprig thyme
- 1 bay leaf
- 1 celery stalk, chopped
- ½ teaspoon nutmeg
- Salt and pepper, to taste

Directions:
1. Cook bacon in an in a medium saucepot for 3-4 minutes.
2. Add butter, carrot, leek, shallot, and celery. Cook for 6-7 minutes or until veggies are tender.
3. Add stock, thyme, bay leaf, chestnuts and bring to boil. Reduce heat and simmer for 25 minutes.
4. Remove from the heat and discard the thyme and bay leaf. Allow to cool slightly and puree using an immersion blender.
5. Reheat the soup and stir in the cream, nutmeg and season to taste. Cook for 5 minutes more. Serve while still hot.

Macros per Serving & Nutrition Facts
- Calories 280
- Total Fat 18 g
- Total Carbohydrate 25 g
- Protein 6 g

# Coconut Mushroom Soup

This soup is made with mushrooms cooked in coconut milk.

Serves: 3
Preparation time: 25 minutes

Ingredients
- 1 cup mushrooms, sliced
- 1 cup coconut milk
- 1 onion, sliced
- 1 cup chicken broth
- 4-5 garlic cloves, minced
- ½ teaspoon black pepper
- ¼ teaspoon salt
- 1 tablespoon oil

Directions
1. Heat oil in a saucepan, add onion and garlic cloves, cook for 1 minute.
2. Add all mushroom and fry for 5 minutes.
3. Add chicken broth, coconut milk, salt, pepper and mix well.
4. Leave to cook on low heat for 15 minutes.
5. Transfer to serving bowls.
6. Serve and enjoy.

Macros per Serving & Nutrition Facts
- Calories 180
- Total Fat 2 g
- Total Carbohydrate 7 g
- Protein 3 g

# Split pea & Quinoa Soup V

There is nothing better than a hearty soup to end the day.

Serves: 4

Time: 1 hour

Ingredients:
- 1 cup yellow split peas
- ½ cup uncooked Quinoa
- cups vegetable broth
- ½ bay leaf
- ¼ teaspoon ground coriander seeds
- ½ tablespoon olive oil
- Salt and pepper, to taste

Directions:
1. Rinse the peas under cold water and remove any black ones.
2. Place the rinsed peas into a saucepan.
3. Add the remaining ingredients and give it a good stir.
4. Cover and cook for 60 minutes. Season to taste and serve while still hot.

Macros per Serving & Nutrition Facts
- Calories 224
- Total Fat 0 g
- Total Carbohydrate 41.8 g
- Protein 13.7 g

## Quinoa and Vegetable soup V

This healthy soup is a combination of quinoa, celery, and smoky flavor coming from the fire roasted tomatoes.

Serves: 8
Time: 50 minutes

Ingredients:
- 8oz. can fire roasted tomatoes
- carrots, diced

- cups vegetable broth
- ¼ teaspoon ground coriander seeds
- 1 tablespoon olive oil
- 8oz. Quinoa uncooked
- 2 celery stalks, chopped
- ¼ teaspoon ground cumin
- Salt and pepper, to taste

Directions:
1. Place all ingredients into a cooker.
2. Stir and set the cooker to simmer.
3. Cook for 45 minutes. Season to taste before serving.

Macros per Serving & Nutrition Facts
- Calories 114
- Total Fat 2 g
- Total Carbohydrate 8 g
- Protein 15 g

# *Mashed & Pureed Foods*

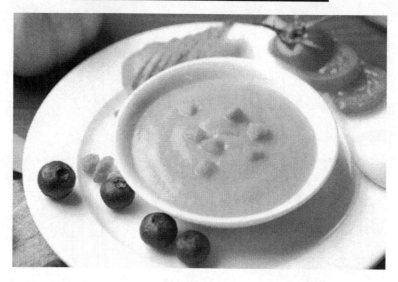

# *Pureed Chicken Noodles with Chicken Thighs 20*

This recipe offers a Chinese flare with pairing noodles with deliciously marinated chicken thighs.

Serving: 3
Time: 15 minutes

Ingredients
- Fresh noodles (24 oz.)
- Garlic (6 cloves, minced)
- Oil (3 Tablespoons)
- Chicken Broth (4 ½ cups)
- Water (1 ½ cups)
- Mushrooms- Shiitake (12, sliced)
- Carrots (12 slices)
- Baby bok choy (12)
- White Pepper (1/4 teaspoon)
- Salt (1/4 teaspoon)
- Chicken Thighs (12 oz., skinless, boneless, cooked, and shredded)

Directions
1. Boil noodles till al dente, then rinse and drain.
2. Put aside till needed. Stir fry garlic in oil till golden, put aside. Heat broth and water then add carrot, mushrooms, bok choy, salt, and pepper to taste. When veggies have cooked, remove from heat.
3. Add chicken noodles in a food processor and process until you have achieved an apple sauce consistency.
4. Serve and top with a dash of garlic oil on top to finish.
Tip: You may also serve with red chili in soy sauce.

Macros per Serving & Nutrition Facts
- Calories 375
- Total Fat 16.3 g
- Total Carbohydrate 36.7 g
- Protein 22.5 g

# Smashed Potato Salad V

This recipe offers the best of both worlds, creamy mashed potatoes with chunks of hard boiled eggs. It's devilishly delicious!

Serves: 6
Time: 35 minutes

Ingredients
- Potatoes (3lbs, Yukon gold, quartered, boiled and mashed)
- Eggs (4 hard boiled, sliced)
- Celery (1 stalk, chopped)
- Radishes (6, thinly sliced)
- Sweet Pickle Relish (2 tbsp.)
- Green Onions (3, thinly sliced)
- Miracle Whip Dressing (3/4 cup)
- Vinegar (1 tbsp., white)
- Paprika (1/2 tsp.)

Directions:
1. Place potatoes while they are still warm into a bowl and add all the remaining ingredients on top then mix until fully combined.
2. Serve and enjoy.

Macros per Serving & Nutrition Facts
- Calories 204
- Total Fat 9 g
- Total Carbohydrate 25 g
- Protein 5 g

# Mashed Roasted Sweet Potato Salad V

Rusty roasted sweet potatoes mixed into a classic potato salad mayonnaise dressing.

Serves: 6
Time: 1 hr and 15 minutes

Ingredients
- Sweet Potatoes (2lbs, chopped and roasted)
- Onion (¼ cup, chopped)
- Green Bell Peppers (1, seeded, and chopped)
- Mixed Vegetable (1 can drained)
- Salt and Pepper (to taste)
- Eggs (3, hard – boiled, chopped)
- Dill (1 tbsp., chopped)
- Mayonnaise (½ Cup)
- Yellow Mustard (1 tsp.)

Directions:
1. Place potatoes while they are still warm into a bowl and add all the remaining ingredients on top then stir until well combined.
2. Add to a food processor and pulse until completely pureed.
3. Serve warm or chilled.

Macros per Serving & Nutrition Facts
- Calories 177
- Total Fat 1 g
- Total Carbohydrate 37.4 g
- Protein 7.5 g

# Pureed Kale Curry

This delight is simply made with blended kale and cooked with the flavors of ginger and garlic.

Serves: 5
Time: 30 minutes

Ingredients:
- cups kale leaves, chopped
- 2 cups chicken broth
- 1 teaspoon garlic paste
- 2-inch ginger sliced, shredded
- ¼ teaspoon turmeric powder
- ¼ teaspoon salt
- 1 green chili
- 1 tablespoon coconut oil
- ½ cup water

Directions
1. In a blender add kale with water and green chili, blend till puree.
2. Now heat oil in a pan and add ginger with garlic, sauté for 1 minute.
3. Add kale and fry for 5 minutes or its color is slightly changed.
4. Pour chicken broth and add salt, leave to cook on low heat for 15-20 minutes.
5. Serve and enjoy.

Macros per Serving & Nutrition Facts
- Calories 269.5
- Total Fat 6.3 g
- Total Carbohydrate 48.5 g
- Protein 7.9 g

## Pureed General Tso's Chicken Thigh

A classic Chinese dish named after a brave General many years ago.

Serving: 2
Time: 30 minutes

Ingredients
- Chicken thigh (10 oz., boneless, skinless, cubed)

- Soy Sauce (1/2 Tablespoon)
- Salt (1/4 teaspoon)
- Cornstarch (1/3 cup)
- Oil (1 Tablespoon)
- Ginger (3 slices, minced)
- Garlic (1 clove, diced)
- Red chilies (5, seeds removed)
- Scallion (2 stalks, white parts)

Sauce

- Chinese rice vinegar (3 Tablespoons)
- Soy sauce (2 ½ Tablespoons)
- Dark soy sauce (1/2 Tablespoon)
- Hoisin sauce (1 teaspoon)
- Water (1/4 cup)
- Cornstarch (1 Tablespoon)

Directions

1. Cover meat in a container with salt and soy sauce; let it marinate for 15 minutes. Mix together the ingredients for the sauce and put aside till needed.
2. Heat oil and put cornstarch on chicken. Cook chicken until browned.
3. Remove from pot with a slotted spoon and place on paper towels to absorb excess oil.
4. Using another pan or wok, heat 1 ½ tablespoons of oil, then add ginger, chilies, and garlic.
5. Cook until chilies are fragrant. Put sauce into wok/pan and cook till sauce gets thick, then add chicken. Stir to combine and add scallions.
6. Add to a food processor and puree until smooth.
7. Serve hot.

Macros per Serving & Nutrition Facts

- Calories 310
- Total Fat 5 g
- Total Carbohydrate 57 g
- Protein 7 g

# *Rustic Pork Ragu Puree*

This amazingly rich Ragu is delicious when paired with noodles, such as pappardelle and fettuccine, but for now, you will can enjoy it with a creamy polenta seeing that will slide right down with the pureed Ragu. Tip: Try the Ragu with Parmesan sprinkled over it.

Serves: 3-4
Time: 2 hours

Ingredients
- Pork (4 lbs.)
- Salt
- Pepper
- Olive Oil (2 Tbsp.)
- Onions (2, large, finely minced)
- Tomato Paste (1/4 Cup)
- Garlic (4 Cloves, minced)
- Lemon Water (1 Cup, Dry)
- Plum Tomatoes, (2 (796ml) Cans, Italian, crushed)
- Star Anise Pods (two)
- Bay Leaf (one)
- Cooked Polenta
- Parmesan Cheese (Shredded)

Directions
1  Trim and discard the excess fat from the top of the roast. Remove the excess liquid from it by patting it dry then proceed to season it with salt and pepper.
2  On medium setting heat the oil in a large Dutch oven. Now, for 3 to 4 minutes per side char the pork, or char it until browned on every side, before transferring it off to a platter.
3  Set your oven to preheat at 250F and as it does, add in your seasoning of onions and tomato paste, occasionally stirring for 10 minutes or until the onion gets very soft. After this,

garlic can be added while continuing to cooking for a minute or two.

4   Add lemon water while stirring and watching for and putting back in any browned bits that are left in the pan. Immediately after, add the crushed tomatoes and tomato juice. Now, put back the roast into the pot and bring the mixture to a boil now by setting the heat to high.

5   The bay leaf and star anise should be wrapped in a cheesecloth pouch, dipped into the sauce and the pot covered. Move the pot now to your preheated oven for cooking for 3 hours. By this time your meat should be tender, falling away from its bone, at which time you may discard the bay leaf and star anise.

6   Remove your meat for cooling for about 5 minutes. Add the pork into a food processor and pulse until completely pureed. Return the pureed pork to the pot, and you may throw out any bone.

7   Serve and enjoy.

Macros per Serving & Nutrition Facts
- Calories 310
- Total Fat 5 g
- Total Carbohydrate 57 g
- Protein 7 g

## *Comforting Chicken Fricassee Puree*

This French stew of chicken and vegetables is a classic; cooked in white wine and with a touch of cream for its finish. The sauce includes tarragon and may even be had by mopping up with bread.

Serves: 3-4
Time: 1 1/2hr

## Ingredients

- Chicken pieces (bones and skin removed, breast halves, drumsticks, thighs, 2 ½ lbs.)
- Salt (¼ tsp)
- Black pepper (add to required taste)
- All-purpose flour (2 tbsp.)
- Olive oil, extra virgin (1 tbsp.)
- Large shallots, finely chopped (5 total, equivalent to 1 cup)
- Lemon water (1 cup)
- Chicken broth (less sodium, 1 ½ cups)
- Carrot, medium, peeled and sliced thin (1)
- Mushrooms, small-button variety, clean and halved or quartered (1 lb.)
- Tarragon (4 sprigs)
- Tarragon, chopped (4 tsp)
- Cornstarch (1 tbsp.)
- Water (1 tbsp.)
- Reduced-fat sour cream (¼ cup)
- Dijon mustard (2 tsp)

## Directions

1. Using salt and pepper season your chicken and dip in flour. Ensure that you shake off any flour excesses before placing it in your Dutch oven or frying pan. Heat and place your chicken to cook until it appears brown for approximately 4 minutes for each side, then move it to a plate when complete.

2. Place your shallots in to cook, and stir for about 30 seconds. Scrape back in any browned bits and include the wine now. Allow to heat for 3 minutes or until they become a bit reduced.

3. The broth should be added and the pot allowed to simmer. Your chicken should be brought back in where you will add mushrooms, tarragon sprigs, and julienne carrots. Lower your heat and cover to simmer until your chicken becomes soft. This process should take approximately 20 minutes, and

you should note that the center of the chicken is no longer pink.

4   Separate the meat from the chicken bone, add to a food processor and process until you achieve a smooth puree. Scoop your chicken puree onto a plate and cover with foil to keep warm. At this time, you may also remove your tarragon sprigs.

5   Set your heat to medium-high to allow the cooking liquid to simmer for 2 or 3 minutes. This last part adds additional flavoring.

6   Cornstarch should now be included in the pot and stirred for 2 minutes until slightly thick. Add some chopped tarragon now, mustard and sour cream.

7   Serve right away, and enjoy.

Macros per Serving & Nutrition Facts
- Calories 250
- Total Fat 5 g
- Total Carbohydrate 27 g
- Protein 24 g

## *Traditional Osso Bucco Puree*

This delicious veal is generally made over a campfire. However today we are making it in our kitchens to be pureed.

Serves: 2-3
Time: 2 hours

Ingredients:
- Rosemary (1 sprig)
- Thyme (1 sprig)
- Bay Leaf (1 dry)
- Cloves (2, whole)
- Cheesecloth
- Kitchen twine

- veal shanks (3, whole, trimmed)
- Sea salt (1 tsp)
- Grounded black pepper (1/2 tsp)
- All-purpose flour (1/2 Cup)
- Vegetable oil (1/2 Cup)
- Onion (1, small, diced)
- Carrot (1, small, diced)
- Celery (1 stalk, diced)
- Tomato Paste (1 Tbsp.)
- Lemon Water (1 Cup)
- Chicken Stock (3 Cups)
- Parsley (3 Tbsp., chopped)
- Lemon Zest (1 Tbsp.)

Directions
1. Create a bouquet garni by tying your cheesecloth with the thyme, rosemary, cloves, and bay leaf cloves inside then secure it with a piece of twine.
2. Use a piece of paper towel to remove the excess moisture from the veal shanks in a patting motion.
3. Next, use another piece of kitchen twine to secure the meat to the bone. Season with salt and pepper then dredge each shank into the flour.
4. Heat the oil in your Dutch oven pot until it begins to smoke. Remove any excess flour and place the veil to brown on all sides.
5. Remove the shanks from the heat and set aside to cool a bit.
6. Once cooled, separate the meat from the veal shank bone and add to a food processor. Process the veal until you achieve a smooth puree (much like an apple sauce texture) and set aside.
7. In the pot, you took the veil from, pour in the carrots, onion, and celery then add salt to season. Sauté for about 8 minutes or until completely soft.

8. Mix in the tomato paste to the carrot mixture in the pot and add browned shank puree. Pour in the lime water and allow it to cook until the liquid is reduced by half.
9. Pour in the 2 cups of the chicken stock along with the bouquet garni and allow boiling.
10. Cover the pot, set the heat to low and simmer until cooked. Ensure that the liquid has not dried out from the puree by checking on it in 15-minute intervals.
11. When the shank puree has cooked remove the puree from the pot and place in preparation to serve.
12. Remove and discard the kitchen twine and the bouquet garni. Use the juices from the pot to pour over the puree.
13. Serve and Enjoy!

Macros per Serving & Nutrition Facts
- Calories 444.8
- Total Fat 10 g
- Total Carbohydrate 11.3 g
- Protein 73.9 g

# *Stewed Pork Puree*

There is nothing like stewed pork from a Dutch pot. Now you can enjoy the meat pureed for easy digestion.

Serves: 3-4
Time: 2 hours

Ingredients
- Thyme (1 sprig)
- Bay Leaf (1 dry)
- Cloves (2, whole)
- Cheesecloth
- Kitchen twine
- Pork (2lbs, trimmed, diced)
- Sea salt (1 tsp)

- Grounded black pepper (1/2 tsp)
- Vegetable oil (1/2 Cup)
- Onion (1, small, diced)
- Carrot (1, small, diced)
- Celery (1 stalk, diced)
- Tomato Paste (1 Tbsp.)
- Lime Water (1 Cup, dry)
- Pork Stock/Chicken Stock (3 Cups)
- Parsley (3 Tbsp., chopped)
- Lemon Zest (1 Tbsp.)

Directions
1. Create a bouquet garni by tying your cheesecloth with the thyme, rosemary, cloves, and bay leaf cloves inside then secure it with a piece of twine.
2. Use a piece of paper towel to remove the excess moisture from the pork pieces in a patting motion. Season with salt and pepper.
3. Heat the oil in your Dutch oven pot until it begins to smoke. Set your pork to brown on all sides. Remove the pork pieces from the heat and set aside.
4. In the pot, you took the pork from, pour in the carrots, onion, and celery then add salt to season.
5. Sauté for about 8 minutes or until completely soft. Mix in the tomato paste to the carrot mixture in the pot and add browned pork.
6. Pour in the lemon water and allow it to cook until the liquid is reduced by half.
7. Pour in the 2 cups of the stock along with the bouquet garni and allow boiling.
8. Cover the pot, set the heat to low and simmer until the meat is literally falling off the bone when lifted.
9. Ensure that the liquid is about ¾ way up the pork by checking on it in 15-minute intervals.
10. When the meat has cooked remove the pork from the pot and add the pork to a food processor. Process the pork until

you achieve a smooth puree then spoon on a plate in preparation to serve.

11. Remove and discard the kitchen twine and the bouquet garni.
12. Use the juices from the pot to pour over the pork puree.
13. Serve and Enjoy!

Macros per Serving & Nutrition Facts
- Calories 300
- Total Fat 13 g
- Total Carbohydrate 6 g
- Protein 34 g

# _Refried Beans_

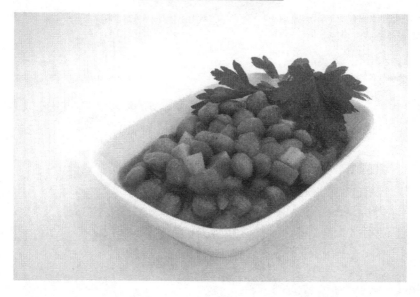

# *Barbecued Baked Beans*

There's no need for meat to make delicious beans!

Serves: 3-4
Time Needed: 1hr

Ingredients
- Yellow Onion (1, chopped)
- Garlic Cloves (5, minced)
- Potatoes (1/4lb., peeled and diced)
- Pinto (1 lb.)
- Water (6 Cups)
- BBQ Sauce (1 Cup)
- Spicy Brown Mustard (2 Tbsp.)
- Adobe Sauce (2 Tbsp., from canned Chipotles)
- Guinness (splash, optional)
- Salt (2 tsp)
- Pepper (1 tsp)

Directions
1. Prepare your beans (wash, sort, and soak) from overnight.
2. Set your Dutch oven to preheat on the top of the stove.
3. Add potatoes to the heated oven and allow to brown. At this point, add onions then proceed to sauté until onions become soft.
4. Continue to sauté while you add the garlic.
5. Continue for about a minute. Pour in the beans, water then cover and allow cooking on low to medium heat for about an hour or until the beans become soft.
6. Add a bit of your preferred BBQ sauce, adobo sauce, mustard salt and pepper while stirring well.
7. Remove the cover and allow simmering until the sauce thickens and the beans become completely cooked (should be about an hour).

Macros per Serving & Nutrition Facts
- Calories 70
- Total Fat 1 g
- Total Carbohydrate 14 g
- Protein 3 g

# *Vegetarian Sweet Potato*

Here is a recipe that will combine a variety of vegetables and beans to get you the same delicious feel of potato going down your palate.

Serves: 5-6
Time: 2 ½ Hours

Ingredients
- Sweet Potato (2 medium, peeled and cut into halves)
- Vegetable Stock (5 Tbsp. 2 Tsp)
- Vegetable oil (2 Tsp each)
- Cocoa (2 Tsp)
- Ground Cumin (2 Tsp)
- Oregano (2 Tsp)
- Salt (2 Tsp)
- Sugar (2 Tsp)
- Onion (1, large)
- Kidney beans (2 Cans)
- Tomatoes (3 Cups, diced, canned)
- Red Bell Pepper (1, diced)
- Yellow Bell Pepper (1, diced)

Directions
1. Set your Dutch oven to preheat over a high flame (350F in in your kitchen) for frying and heat oil.
2. Set the Potato in the heated oil to brown. Stir in onion and allow frying until it appears to be clear.

3. Excluding the kidney beans, and everything else to the pot and reduce heat (225F if in your kitchen).  Cover and simmer for about an hour.
4. Remove cover, add kidney beans and allow simmering as is for an hour. Serve and Enjoy!

Macros per Serving & Nutrition Facts
- Calories 230.7
- Total Fat 3.4 g
- Total Carbohydrate 45.8 g
- Protein 12 g

# *Smoky Barbecue Beans*

When planning to serve slow smoked meats, the best accompaniment you can get for them is fresh homemade beans. The best part is that these beans are not hard to make and very delicious.

Serves: 3-4
Time: 1 hr

Ingredients:
- Vegetarian Bacon (center cut, 5 slices, chopped)
- Yellow Onion (1, chopped)
- Garlic Cloves (5, minced)
- Pinto (1 lb.)
- Water (6 Cups)
- BBQ Sauce (1 Cup)
- Spicy Brown Mustard (2 Tbsp.)
- Adobe Sauce (2 Tbsp., from canned Chipotles)
- Guinness (splash, optional)
- Salt (2 Tsp)
- Pepper (1 tsp)

Directions

1. Prepare your beans (wash, sort, and soak) from overnight.
2. Set your Dutch oven to preheat on the top of the stove. Add bacon to the heated oven and allow to brown until crisp.
3. At this point, add onions then proceed to sauté until onions become soft.
4. Continue to sauté while you add the garlic. Continue for about a minute. Pour in the beans, and water then cover and allow cooking on low to medium heat for about an hour or until the beans become soft.
5. Add a bit of your preferred BBQ sauce along with the brown sugar, adobo sauce, mustard salt and pepper while stirring well.
6. Remove the cover and allow simmering until the sauce thickens and the beans become completely cooked (should be about an hour).
7. Serve and enjoy.

Macros per Serving & Nutrition Facts

- Calories 210
- Total Fat 1.5 g
- Total Carbohydrate 41 g
- Protein 8 g

# Conclusion

There you have it! Together we have explored 50 Amazingly Simple Recipes that you can enjoy within Stage 2 of recovery from a Gastric Sleeve Surgery. We hope you will consider joining us again when we explore the remaining two stages of post operation diet procedures. Achieving a speedy and successful recovery is vital right now, and we want to help you get there. See you next time.